EVERYONE

SMILES!

Ashley N. Grisham & Gary L. Kersey, Jr.

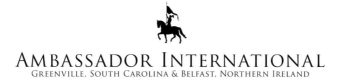

Ambassador International

GREENVILLE, SOUTH CAROLINA & BELFAST, NORTHERN IRELAND

www.ambassador-international.com

Everyone Smiles!

ISBN: 978-1-62020-510-5
eISBN:978-1-62020-415-3

Page Layout: Hannah Nichols
Ebook Conversion: Anna Riebe Raats

Photographs used with permission, courtesy of:
Hannah Nichols Photography
The Sweetest Things Photography
Kristin Burke Photography

AMBASSADOR INTERNATIONAL
Emerald House
427 Wade Hampton Blvd
Greenville, SC 29609, USA
www.ambassador-international.com

AMBASSADOR BOOKS
The Mount
2 Woodstock Link
Belfast, BT6 8DD, Northern Ireland, UK
www.ambassadormedia.co.uk

The colophon is a trademark of Ambassador

In Dedication To All Those Who Brighten Our SMILES

Parents: Dr. Milton "Joe" and Michelle Grisham,
Gary and Cyndi Kersey

Siblings: Alanah Grisham and Sheraz Wiley

The Boys & Girls Clubs of America

The Children of the Shanghai Healing Home

Charles and Omega Collins, Geraldine "Mimi" Grisham,
and Miss Jordyn Jennings

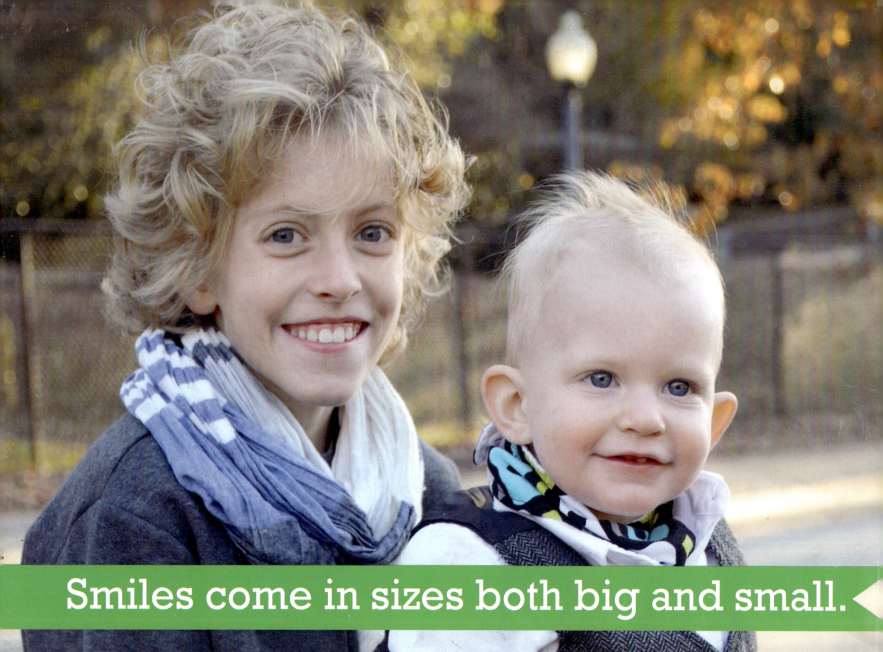

Smiles come in sizes both big and small.

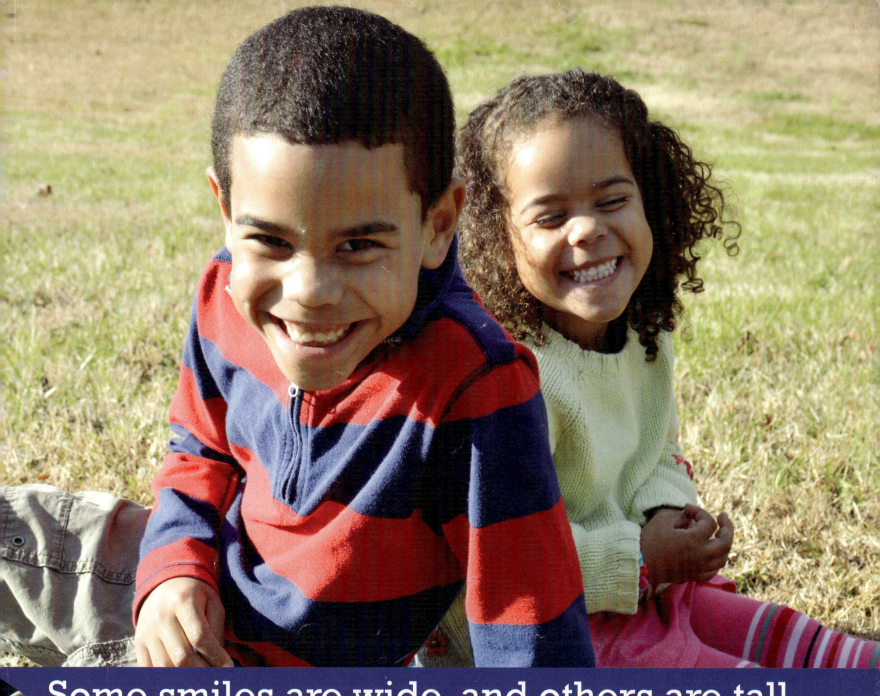

Some smiles are wide, and others are tall.

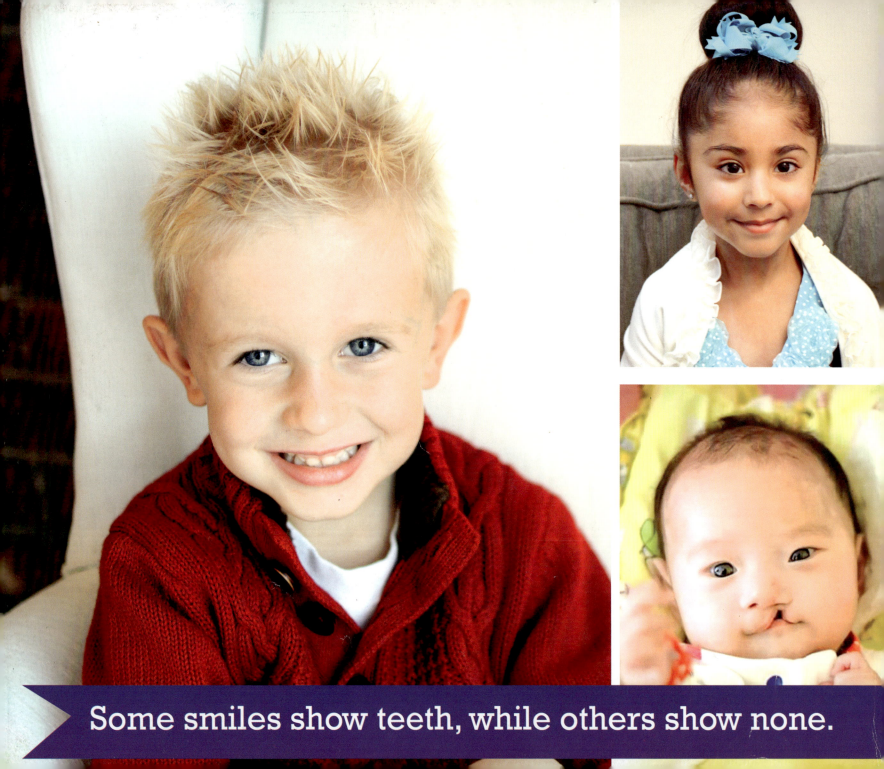

Some smiles show teeth, while others show none.

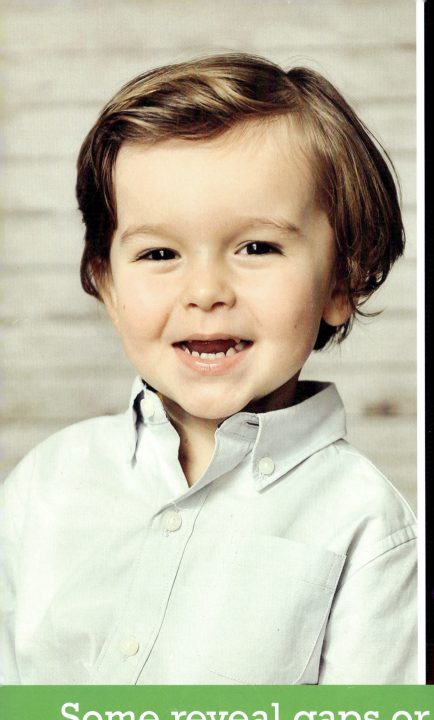
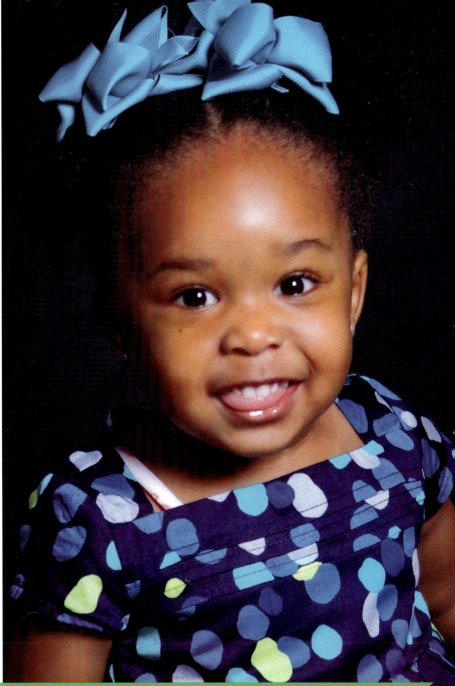

Some reveal gaps or the tip of a tongue.

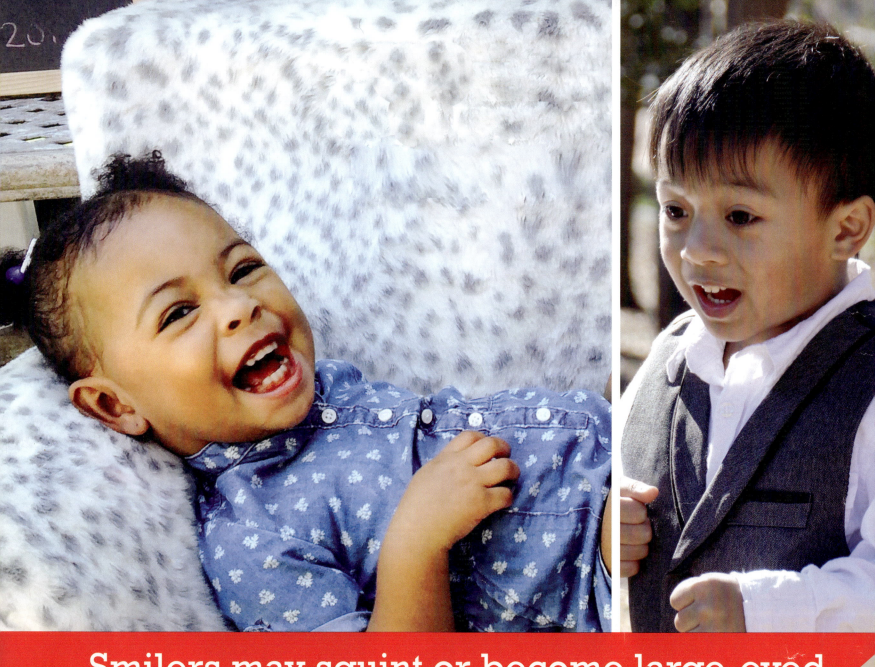

Smilers may squint or become large-eyed,

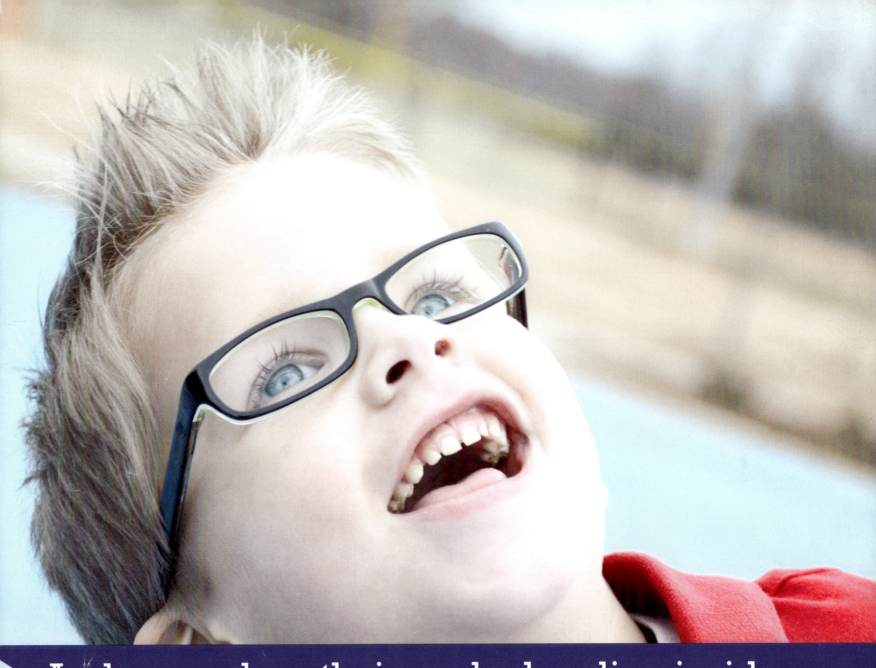

And some show their uvula dangling inside.

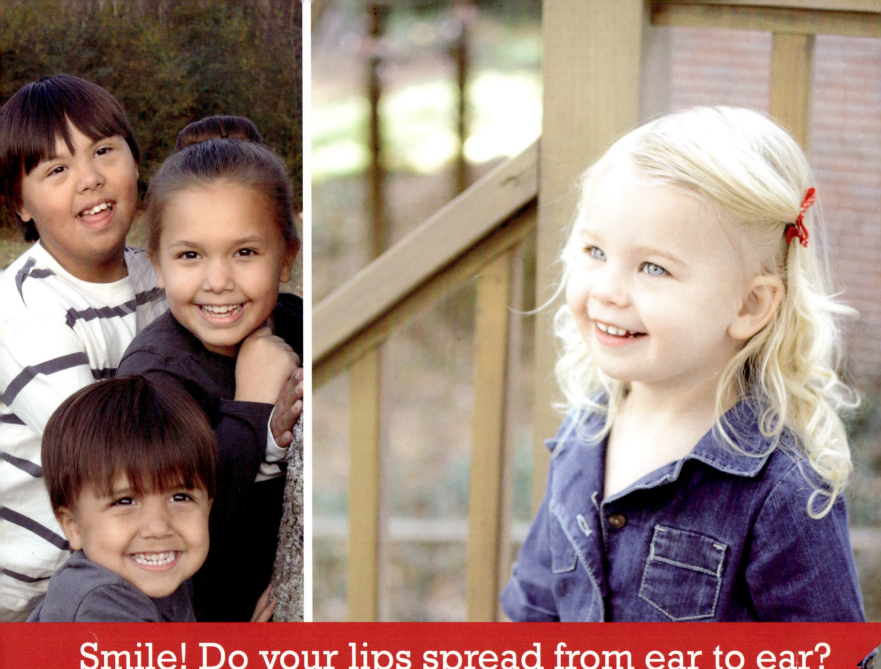

Smile! Do your lips spread from ear to ear?

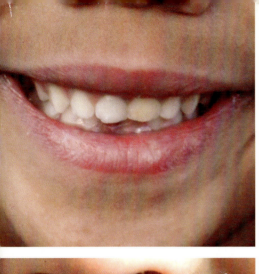
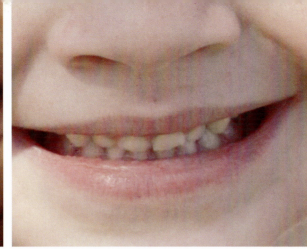
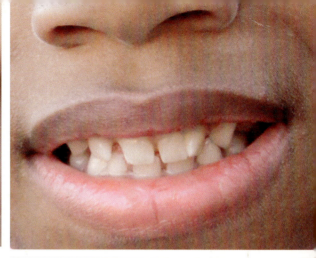

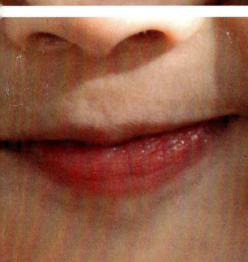

Point to your smile if your smile is shown here.

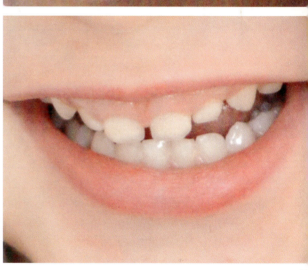

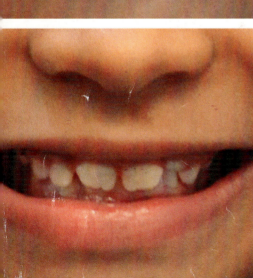
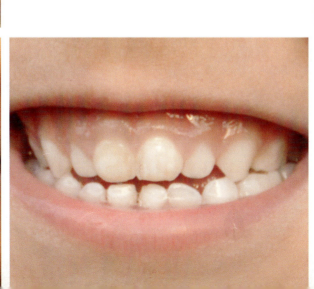
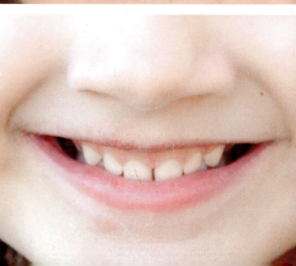

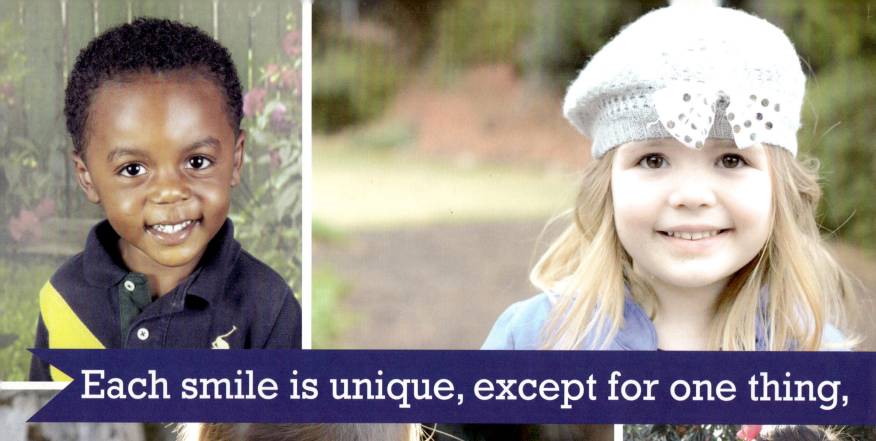

Each smile is unique, except for one thing,

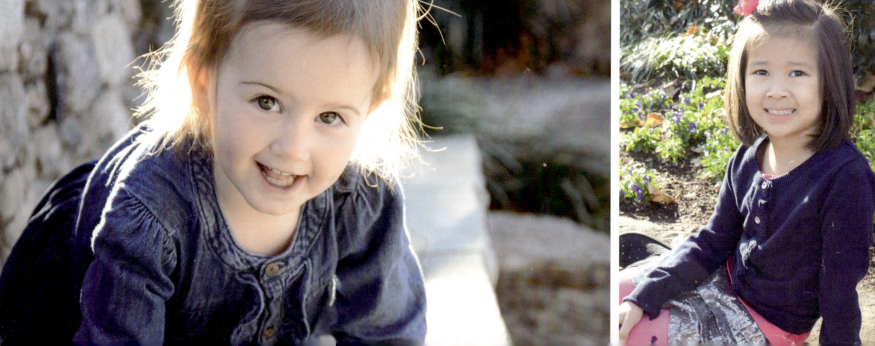

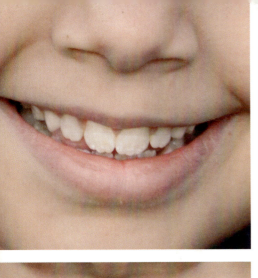
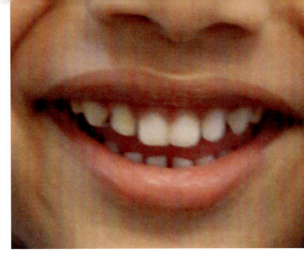
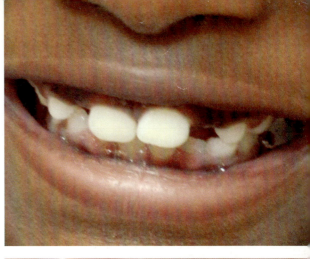
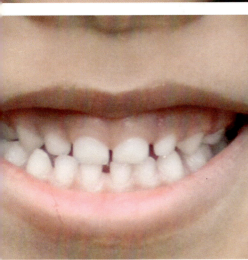

If you look inside, all smiles have teeth!

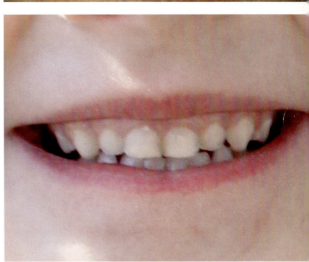
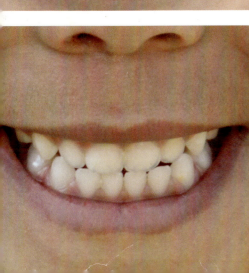
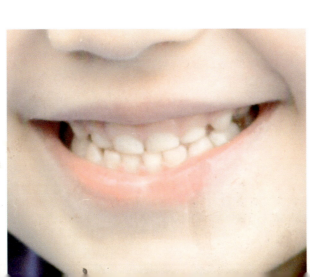
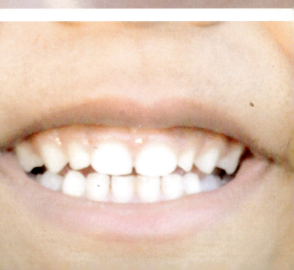

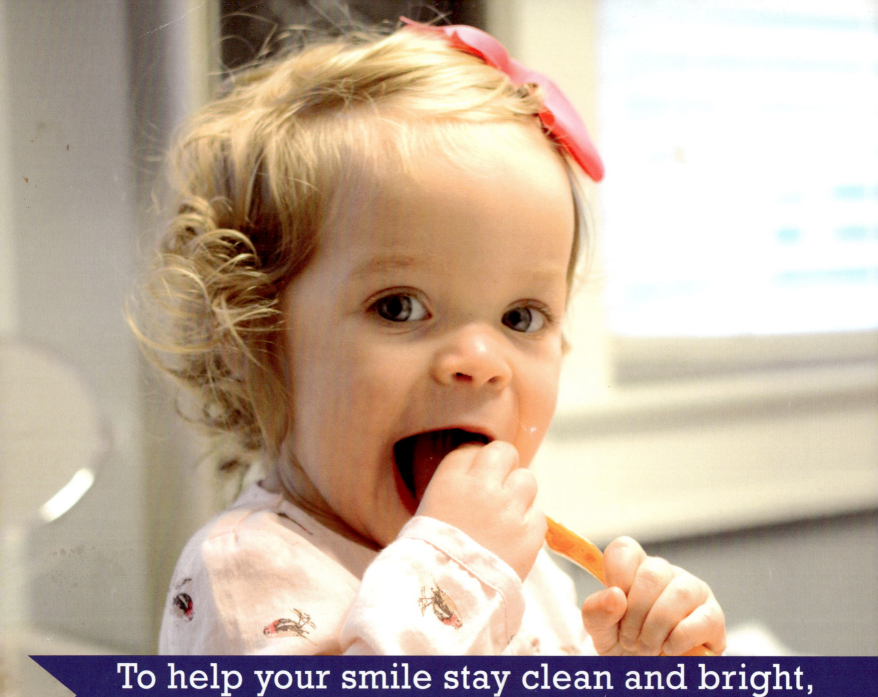

To help your smile stay clean and bright,
Please brush your teeth both morning and night.

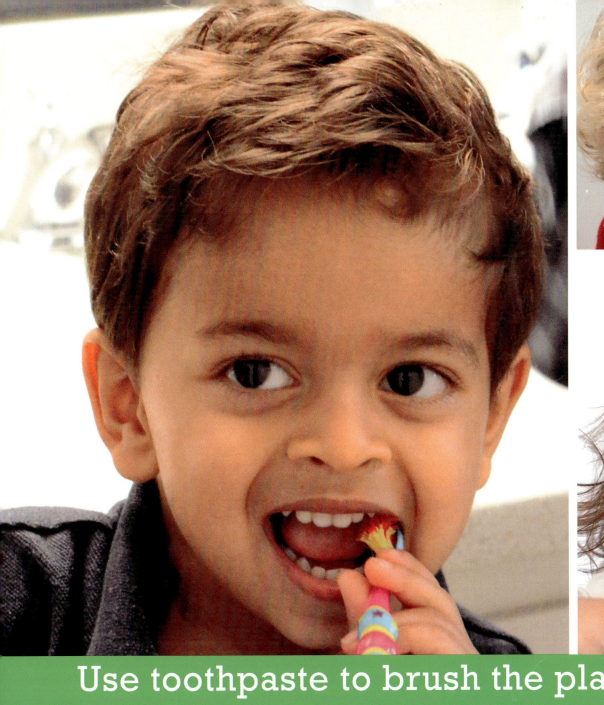
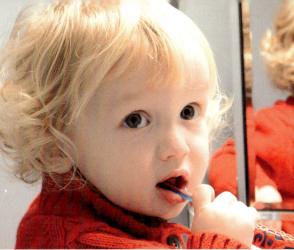
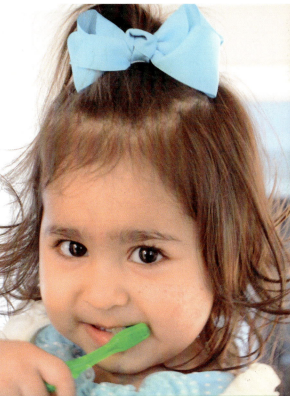

Use toothpaste to brush the plaque away.
Brushing helps fight cavities every day.

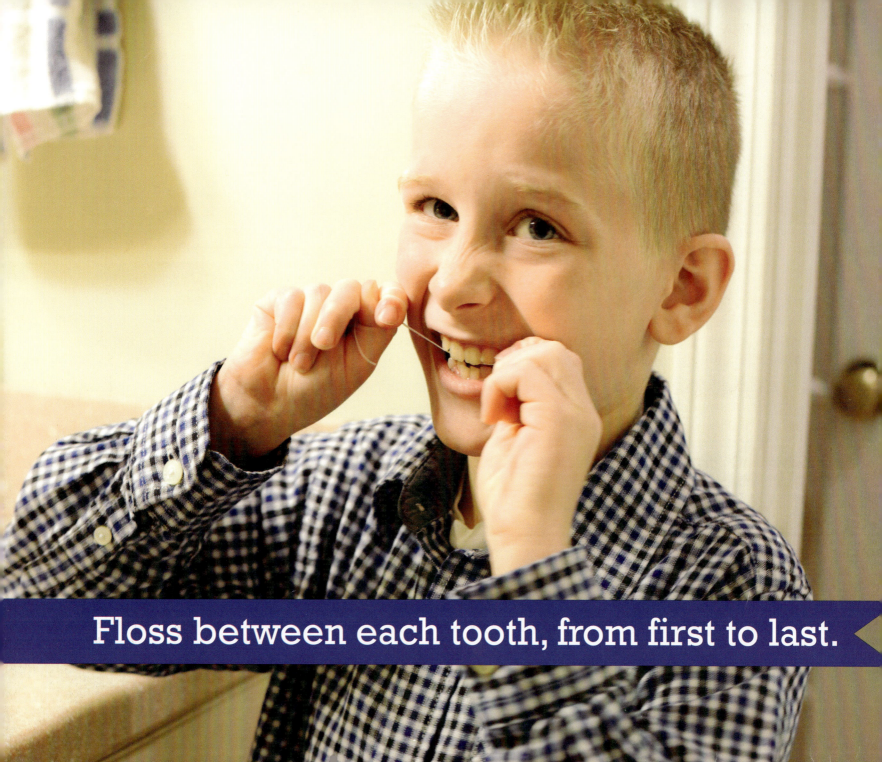

Floss between each tooth, from first to last.

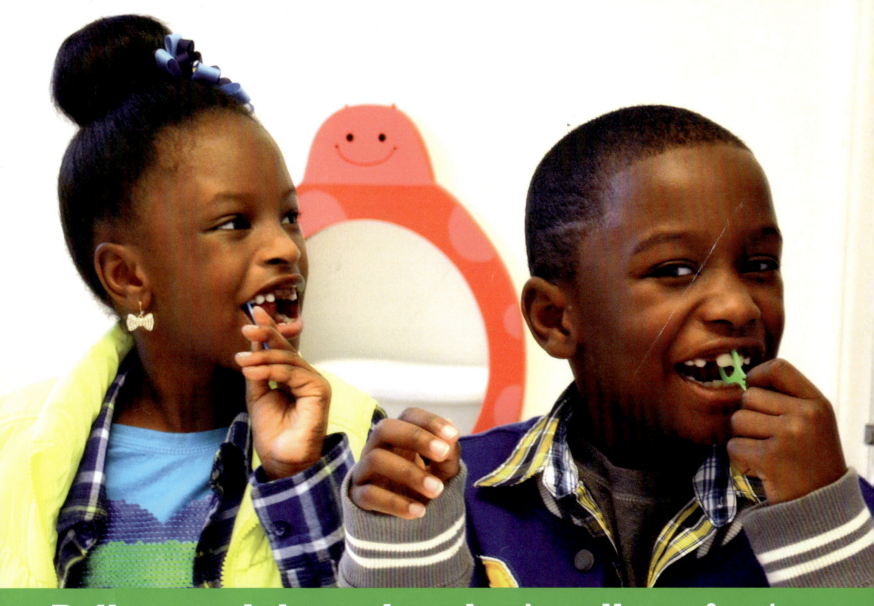

Pull up and down, but don't pull too fast!

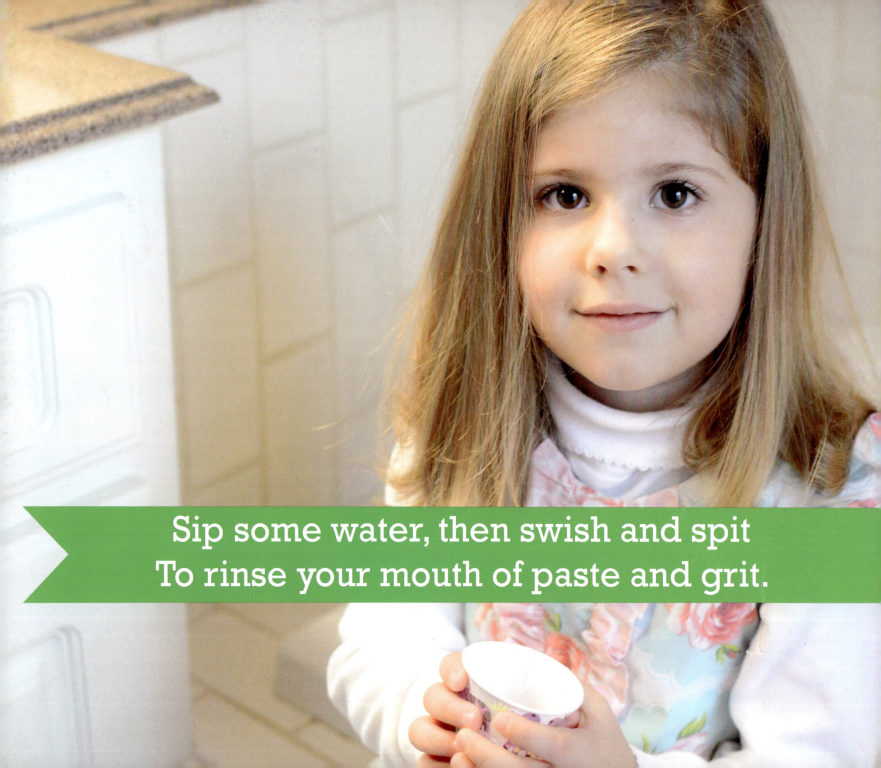

Sip some water, then swish and spit
To rinse your mouth of paste and grit.

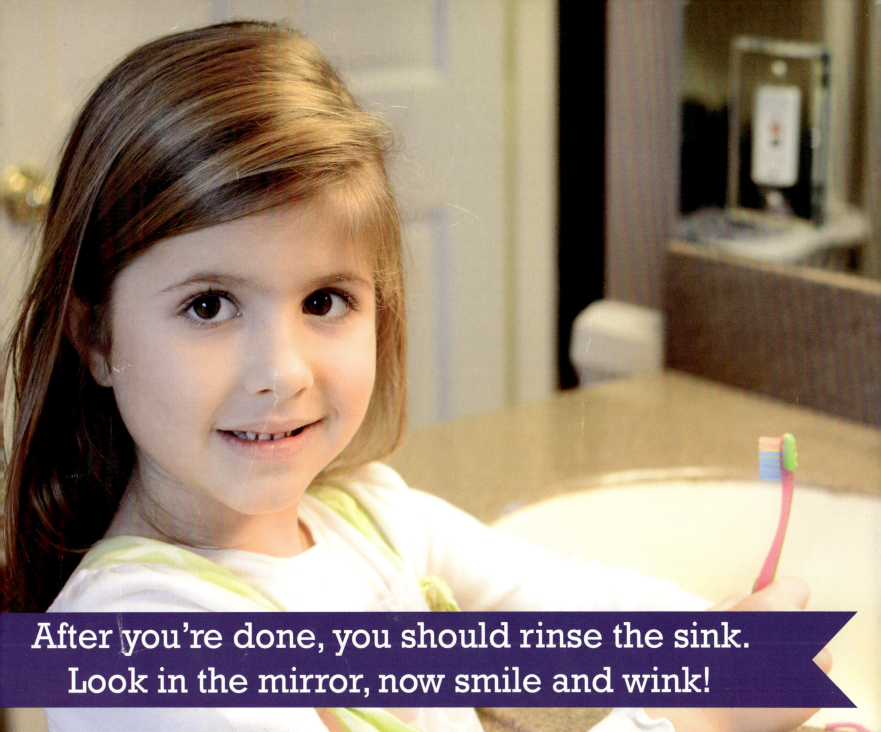

After you're done, you should rinse the sink.
Look in the mirror, now smile and wink!

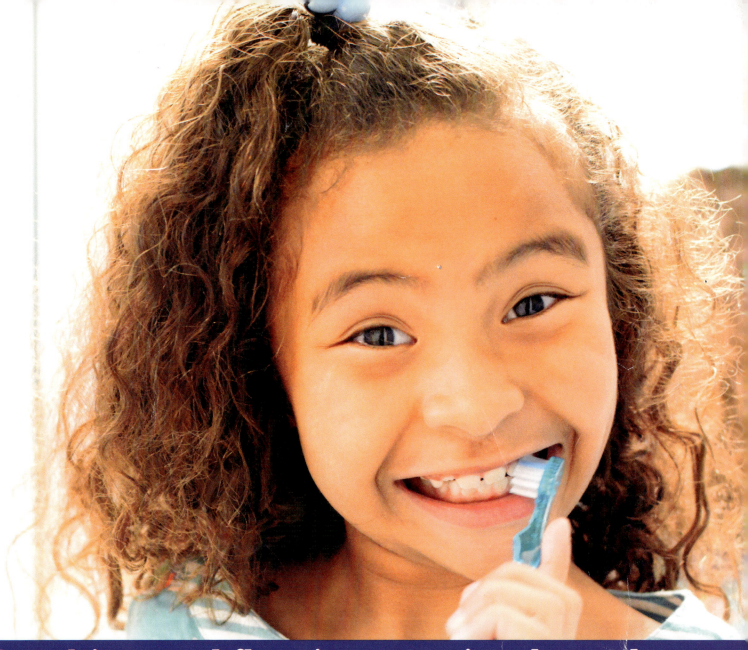

Brushing and flossing are simple to do.
Take care of your teeth, and they'll take care of you.

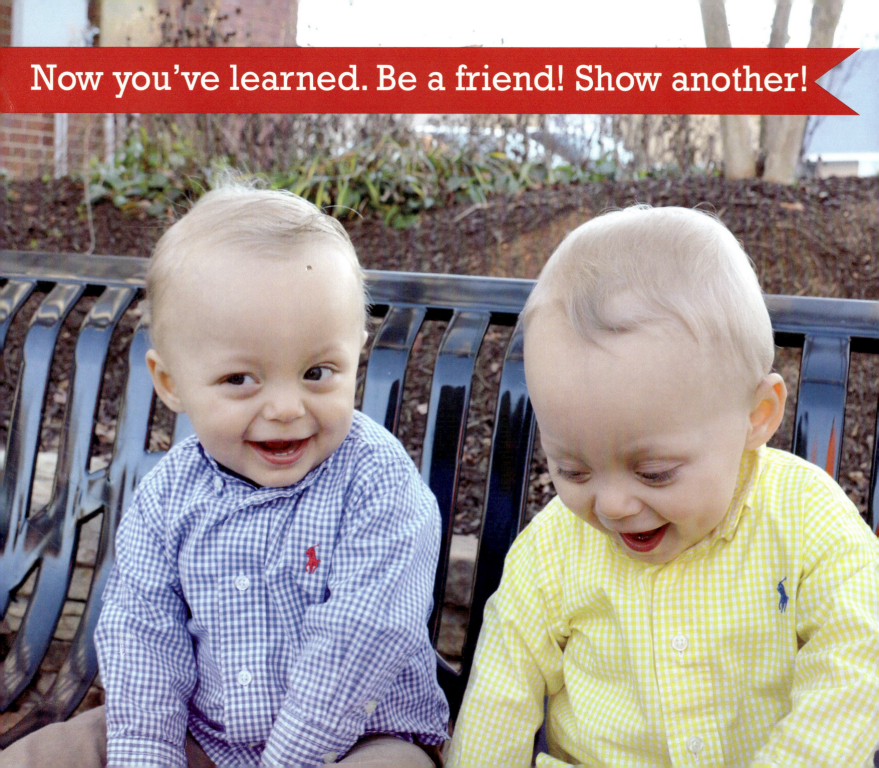

Now you've learned. Be a friend! Show another!

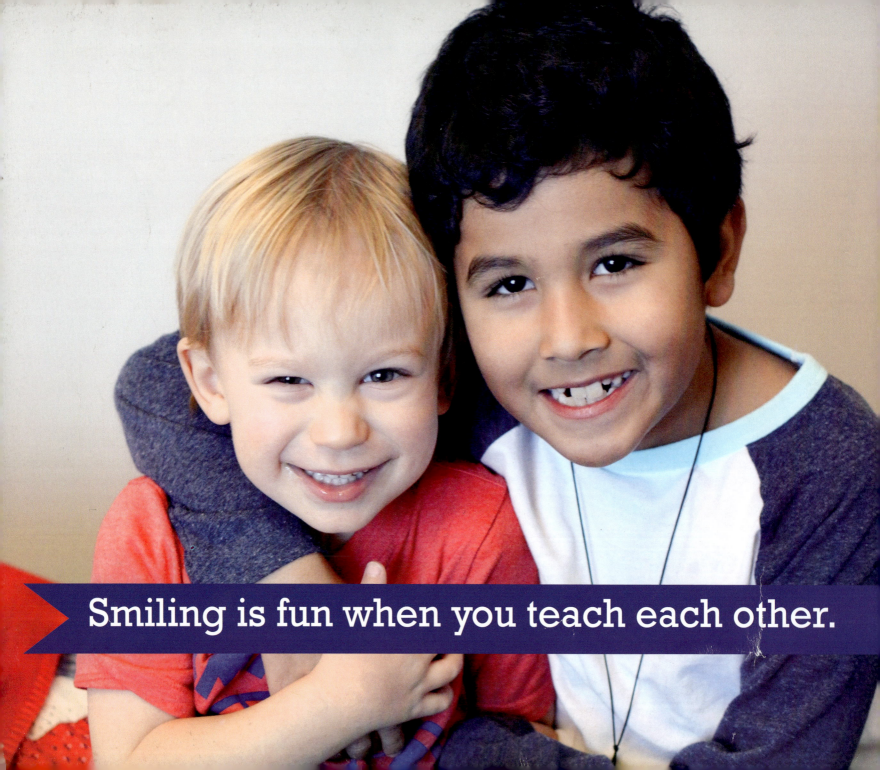

Smiling is fun when you teach each other.

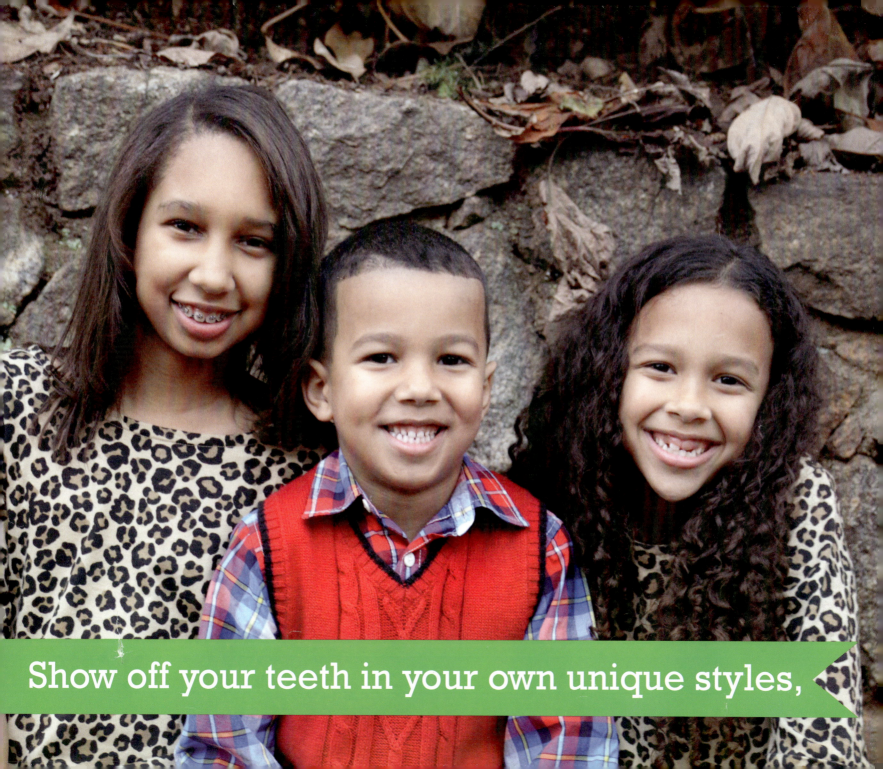

Show off your teeth in your own unique styles,

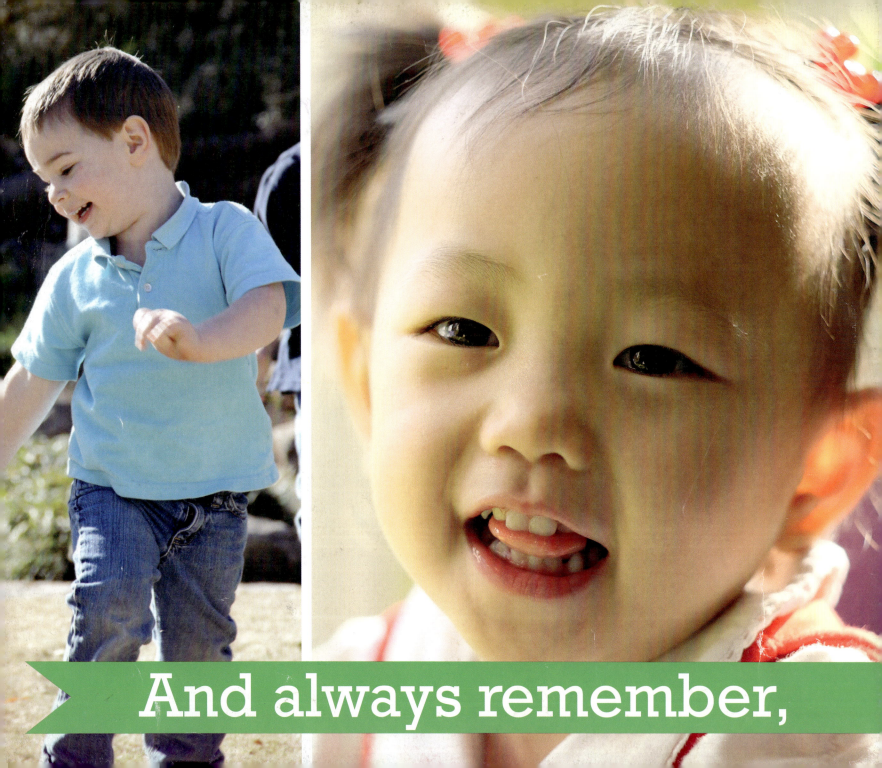

And always remember,

Everyone Smiles!

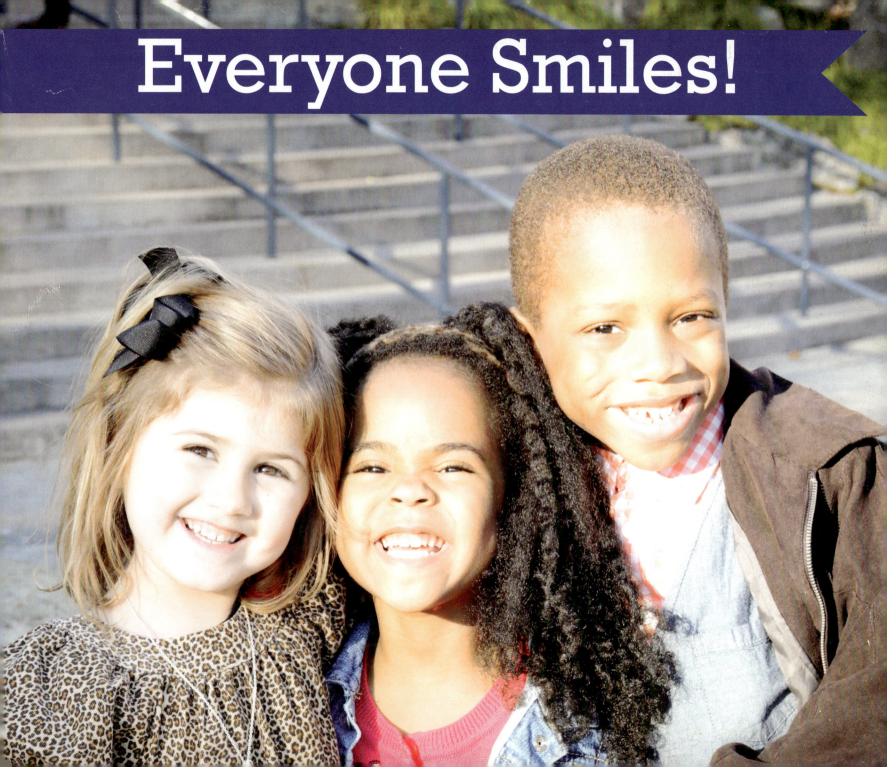

Gary L. Kersey, Jr.

Gary earned his undergraduate degree with honors from Morehouse College where he studied Spanish and minored in Biology. After completing his undergraduate studies, he continued his education by working towards a Masters degree in Physiology & Biophysics from Georgetown University with a focus on Complementary and Alternative Medicine. Gary is an aspiring dental professional and is currently applying to dental school. He hopes to combine his background in the sciences and modern languages to elevate dental care in underserved areas. Gary was born and raised in North Carolina. In his spare time, Gary enjoys tennis, basketball, cooking, volunteering, and traveling.

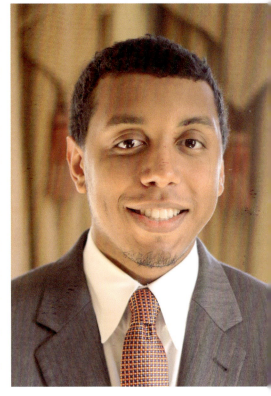

For more information about
EVERYONE SMILES
please visit:

www.everyonesmilesbook.com

every1smiles.book@gmail.com

Ashley N. Grisham

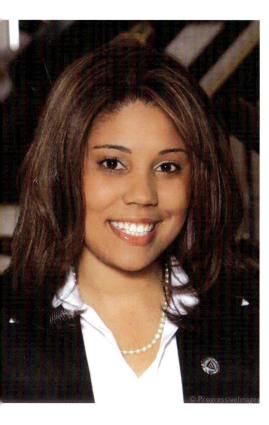

Ashley, a native of San Diego, CA, grew up as the daughter of both a U.S. Navy Captain dentist and a dental hygienist. *Everyone Smiles* was inspired by Grisham's travels all around the world, where she interacted with children who often broke the language and cultural barrier with a smile. A graduate of Spelman College, Grisham earned her Bachelor of Arts in International Studies and holds a minor in Chinese language. Ashley is currently finishing her last year at Georgetown law school and upon graduation will join the law firm of Paul Hastings LLP. In her free time Ashley enjoys kayaking, musical theatre, serving as a creative consultant & playing with her dog Bella.

For more information about
AMBASSADOR INTERNATIONAL
please visit:

www.ambassador-international.com

@AmbassadorIntl

www.facebook.com/AmbassadorIntl

Special Thanks

Dr. Lerita Coleman-Brown

Aureller Cabiness

Dr. Ford Cooper

Dr. Lori Dominguez-Rucker

Erin Ellis

Ann Ennis

Dr. Francisco Ramos-Gomez

Kenneth Green

SaMya Griffin

Mahogany Hanks

Kiara Hill

Dr. Jeanette Holloway

Dr. Douglas Rucker

Mr. Ajit Samarasinghe

Dean David Taylor

Dr. Don Timpton

Our Alma Maters Spelman and Morehouse College

Proverbs 31:25 | Ephesians 6:7